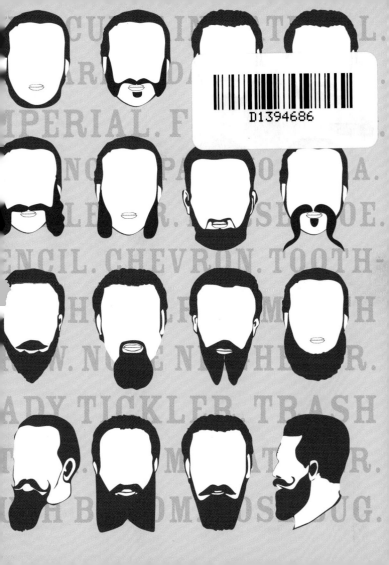

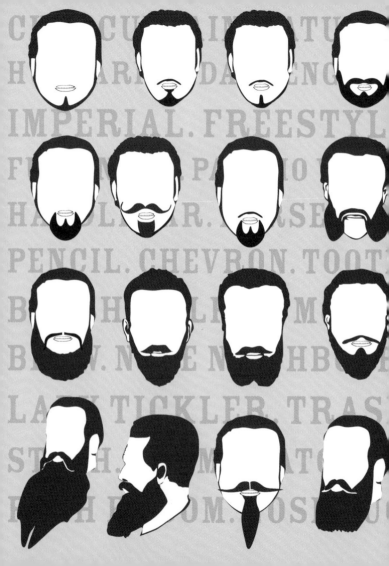

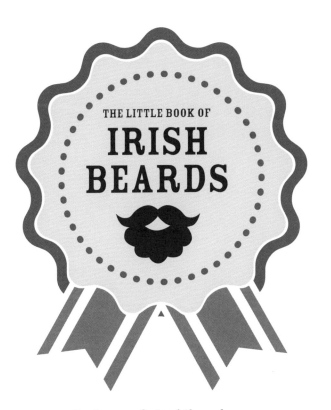

THE LITTLE BOOK OF

IRISH
BEARDS

Barba non facit philosophum
A beard does not constitute a philosopher

… we beg to differ

First published 2015 by The O'Brien Press Ltd
12 Terenure Road East, Rathgar, Dublin 6, Ireland, D06 HD27
Tel: +353 1 4923333; Fax: +353 1 4922777
E-mail: books@obrien.ie
Website: www.obrien.ie

ISBN: 978-1-84717-792-6

1 3 5 7 8 6 4 2
15 17 19 20 18 16

Images courtesy of: Shutterstock (front and back cover photographs, beard icons, hair-dressing icons, Victorian gentleman, Victorian frame, Jamie Dornan); Rexfeatures (The Dubliners, Phil Lynott, Shane Lynch, James Joyce, George Bernard Shaw, Bram Stoker, Roger Casement, George Best); Photocall (Marty Whelan, Brendan Grace, Willie O'Dea, David Norris, Gerry Adams); Sportsfile (John Aldridge, Barry McGuigan, Darren Clarke, Gordon D'Arcy, Colm Parkinson, Conor McGregor, Eoin 'The Bomber' Liston) & Kilmainham Gaol (John MacBride).

Printed and bound in Poland by Białostockie Zakłady Graficzne S.A.

THE LITTLE BOOK OF
IRISH
BEARDS

THE FIVE O'CLOCK SHADOWS

THE O'BRIEN PRESS
DUBLIN

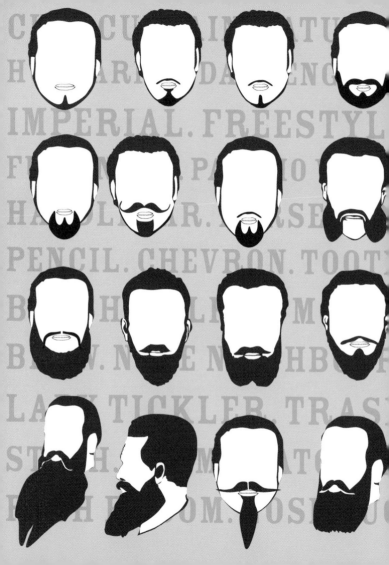

CONTENTS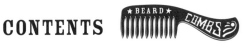

BEARDED HALL
OF FAME RATINGS

In our capacity as judges of all things beard,
we have awarded 'whiskers', as follows:

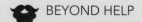 BEYOND HELP

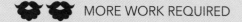 MORE WORK REQUIRED

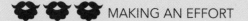 MAKING AN EFFORT

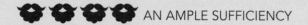 AN AMPLE SUFFICIENCY

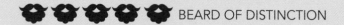 BEARD OF DISTINCTION

❧ INTRODUCTION

We've all seen them, those splendid individuals with various tufts and waves sprouting from their faces like coiffured poodles, those proud wearers of the beard. Whether you spot them in a bike shop discussing the merits of the fixed-wheel bicycle or enjoying an IPA at a nearby craft brewery, these hirsute folk are unavoidable.

However the celebration of the 'lip sweater' is by no means a new event; over the years and centuries, many a famous – or infamous – Irishman has sported some sort of furry arrangement about the face, from the heavy 'chin curtains' of the Victorians to the 'five o'clock shadows' of many who just aren't trying!

This little book aims to celebrate the bearded amongst us, by taking a look at these gentlemen and their bewhiskered visages. We also feel, given the spectacular quality of some of the specimens, that 'whisker' ratings should be awarded throughout. The genii that inhabit these pages are known for their exploits in other fields – winning Nobel Prizes, running the country, or exhibiting sporting prowess – but we feel they *really* should be looked at for the fecundity of their beards.

So sit back, relax and enjoy the celebration of the Irish Beard!

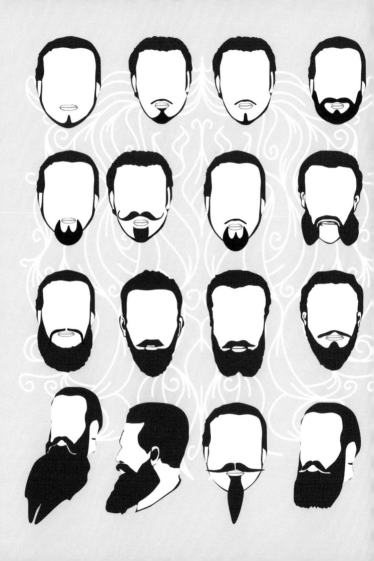

BEARDS

of

HISTORY

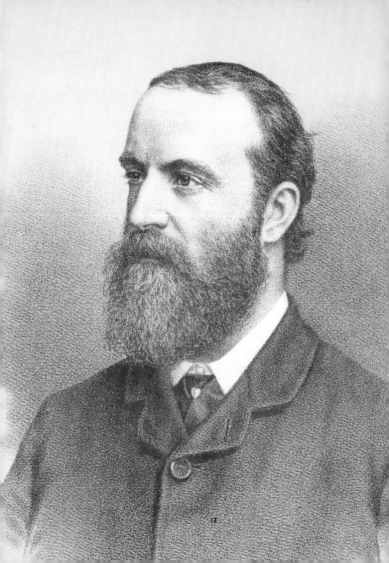

14

CHARLES STEWART PARNELL

The dashing Charles Stewart Parnell is as well
known for his red-hot affair with Kitty O'Shea
(who no doubt simply couldn't resist that
Victorian beard) as for his Home Rule politics.

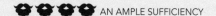 AN AMPLE SUFFICIENCY

❧ HUGH O'NEILL

This Gaelic lord is best known for leading the resistance during the Nine Years' War. We are sure that the combination of tache, beard and steely-eyed gaze put the fear of God into every person who ever crossed his path.

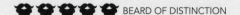 BEARD OF DISTINCTION

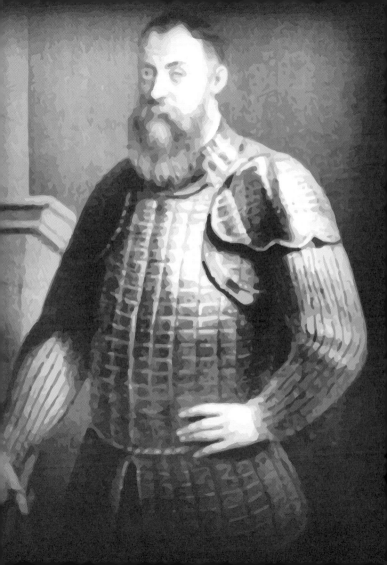

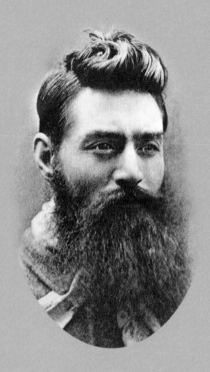

NED KELLY

This notorious outlaw, of Irish extraction, led something of a (no pun intended) hairy life. He and his band of furry-faced associates rampaged across Australia until his final showdown with the law in 1880. He's the subject of more biographies than any other Australian, and is it any wonder with facial arrangements such as these?

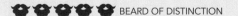 BEARD OF DISTINCTION

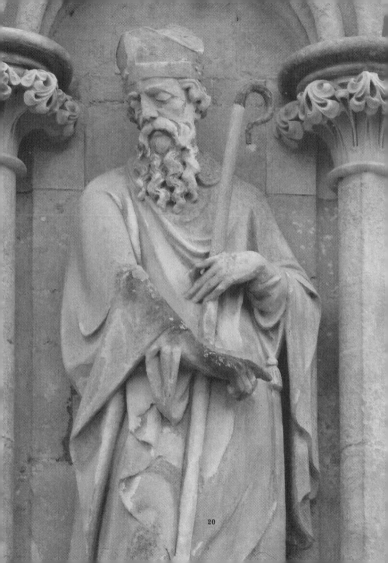

20

🐑 SAINT PATRICK

'Hail glorious Saint Patrick, sweet saint of our isle ...' The most famous Irishman ever to be born in Wales ... And wasn't he great? He brought us Christianity and rid us of snakes, even though in every depiction we see of him you'd have to wonder if said snakes made it into his beard?

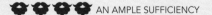

🐑 🐑 🐑 🐑 AN AMPLE SUFFICIENCY

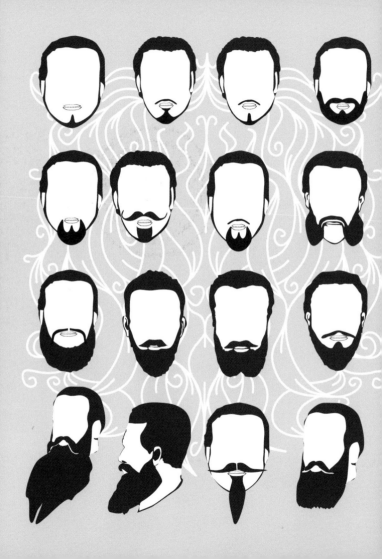

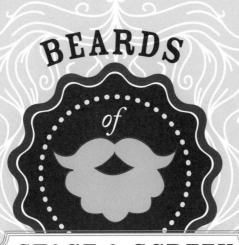

BEARDS

of

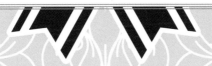

• STAGE & SCREEN •

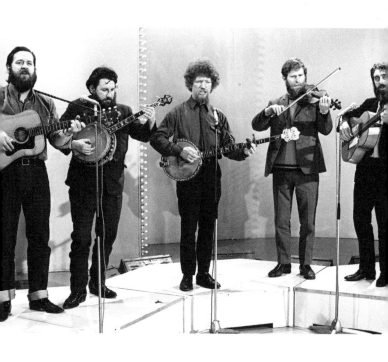

❧ THE DUBLINERS

What's the collective noun for a group
of bearded musicians? It could well be 'A
Dubliners'! Ireland's favourite folk band is a
veritable thicket of beards; perhaps 'twas their
mighty facial fur that gave strength and character
to their voices.

BEARD OF DISTINCTION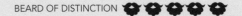

PHIL LYNOTT

Lead singer of Thin Lizzy, Phil not only sported
a chaotic afro on his beautiful head, but was one of
very few males who could carry off a ronnie.
Ireland's coolest rock star – ever!

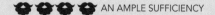 AN AMPLE SUFFICIENCY

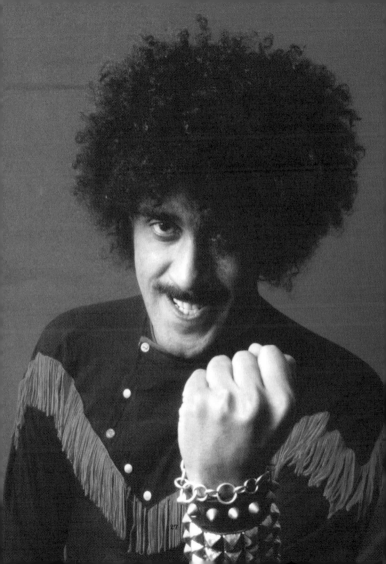

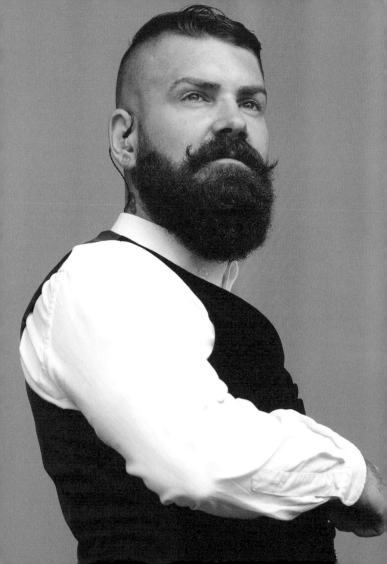

SHANE LYNCH

'Love me for a reason,' sang/mimed Shane Lynch
in his Boyzone days. Well, this fantastic face-
warmer has certainly given us one; it's a beaut!

BEARD OF DISTINCTION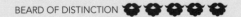

MARTY WHELAN

Ireland's answer to Tom Selleck, all hail Marty,
King of the Moustache!

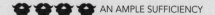 AN AMPLE SUFFICIENCY

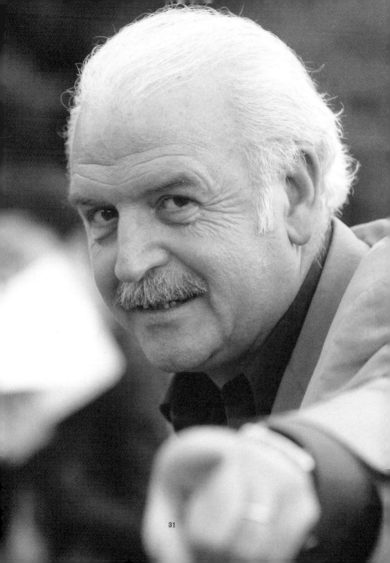

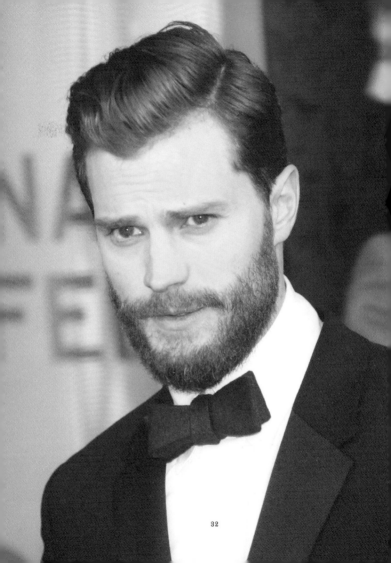

JAMIE DORNAN

Jamie's most famous acting role must be that of notorious King of BDSM; Christian Grey in the *Fifty Shades* saga. It's a pity that he couldn't keep his chin-tickler for the part – who knows what effect it could have had on his leading lady.

BEARD OF DISTINCTION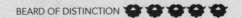

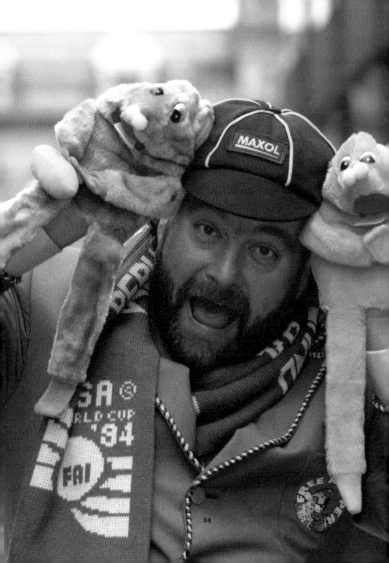

❧ BRENDAN GRACE

In the 1980s Brendan Grace was most famous for his humanitarian work, liberating the oppressed Nipper population (pictured) from their captivity in Ireland's petrol stations. Since then, he's spent some time on Craggy Island. Was this the best beard Fr Ted had ever seen? Well, that would be an ecumenical matter.

 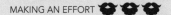

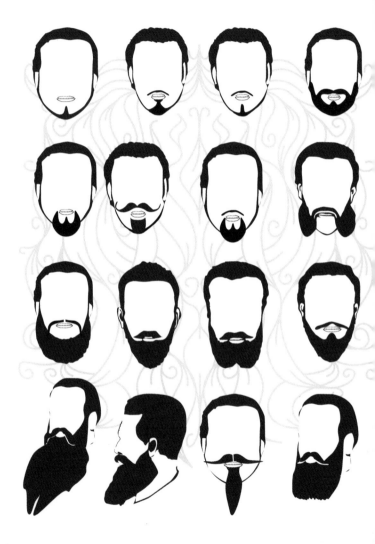

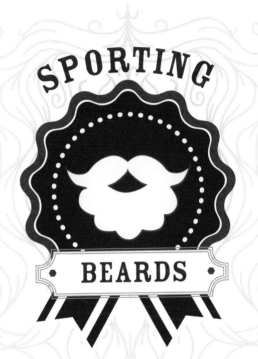

🫘 GEORGE BEST

What is better looking than George Best?

George Best with a beard!

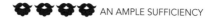 AN AMPLE SUFFICIENCY

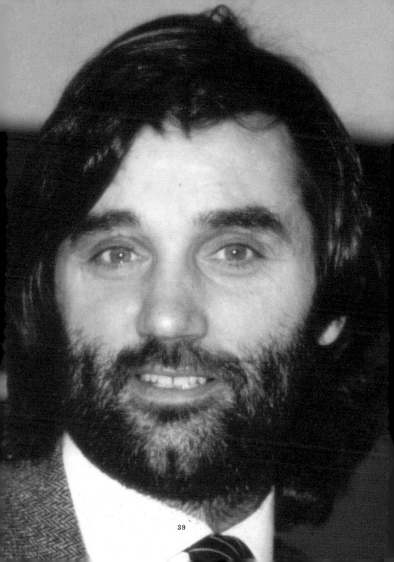

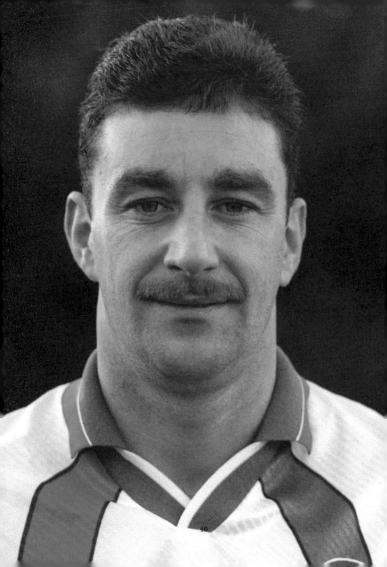

JOHN ALDRIDGE

What's that Scouser doing in the book?! Well, the 'Granny Rule' got him on the team, his performances won him a place in our hearts and that lip-rug got him in the book! Calm down, calm down!

MAKING AN EFFORT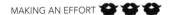

🐾BARRY MCGUIGAN

Known by most as the Clones Cyclone, this boxing legend will always be the Monaghan Moustache to us. A cracking lip-tickler!

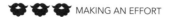 MAKING AN EFFORT

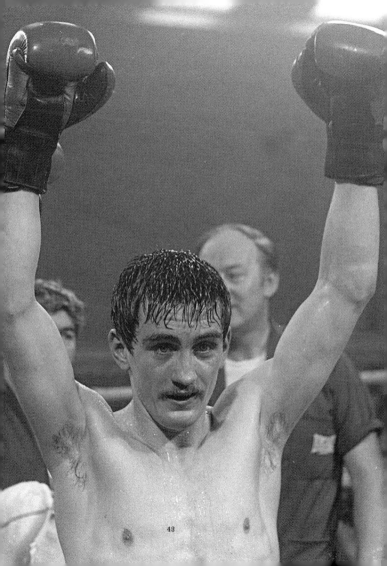

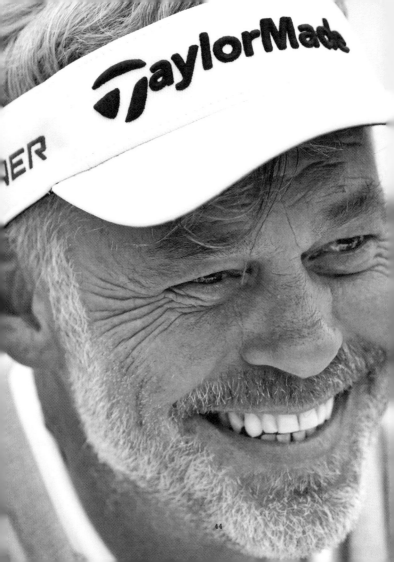

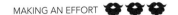 DARREN CLARKE

Golf is not renowned as the trendiest of sports, but with that dashing beard, dapper Darren Clarke will have the hipsters swinging their clubs before you can say 'craft beer'.

MAKING AN EFFORT

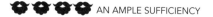 GORDON D'ARCY

Gordon D'Arcy has a beard so strong he uses it to clean his boots after winning a Grand Slam.

AN AMPLE SUFFICIENCY

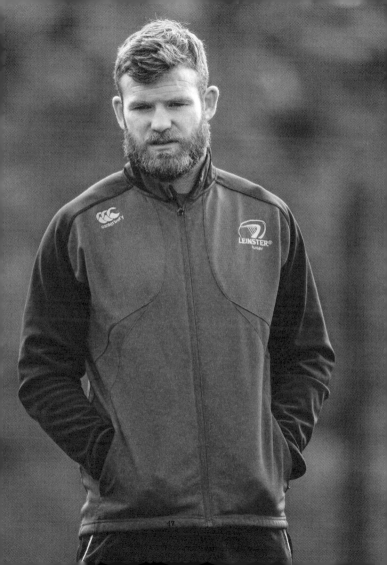

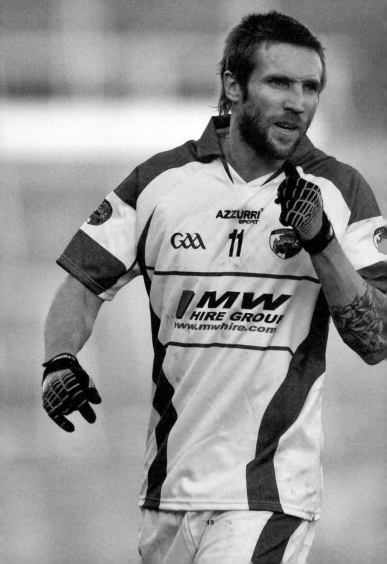

❧ COLM 'WOOLY' PARKINSON

This former Laois player may be 'wooly' by name, but he is certainly no sheep! Famed for speaking his mind on Newstalk's 'Off the Ball', we prefer to honour him for his fantastic facial hair (and give an honourable mention to his BA in Finance).

AN AMPLE SUFFICIENCY ❧ ❧ ❧ ❧

CONOR MCGREGOR

The Notorious Conor McGregor is a Mixed
Martial Arts and Ultimate Fighting Champion,
but to us he'll always be the UFC – Ultimate
Furry Chin.

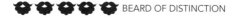 BEARD OF DISTINCTION

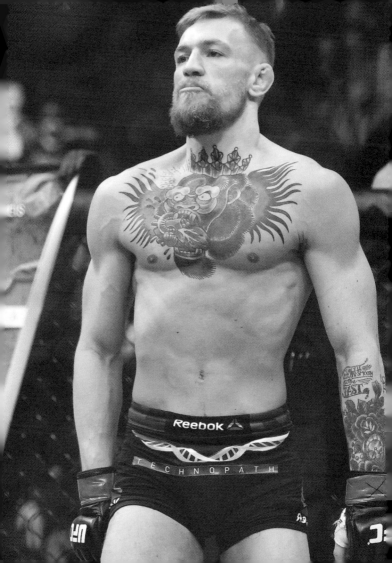

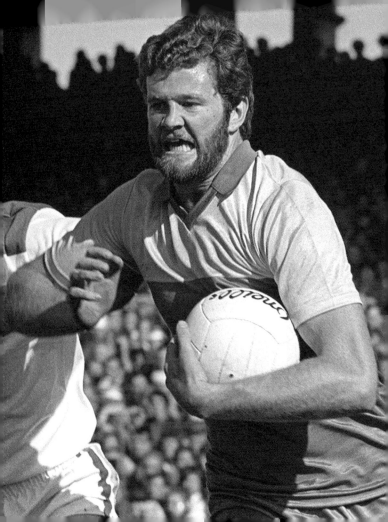

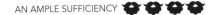 EOIN 'THE BOMBER' LISTON

Ballybunion wouldn't be renowned for blazing
a fashion trail, but 'The Bomber' Liston was
sporting a fine beard the first time vinyl was cool.

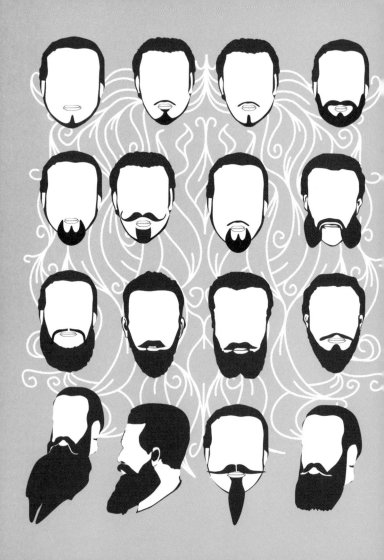

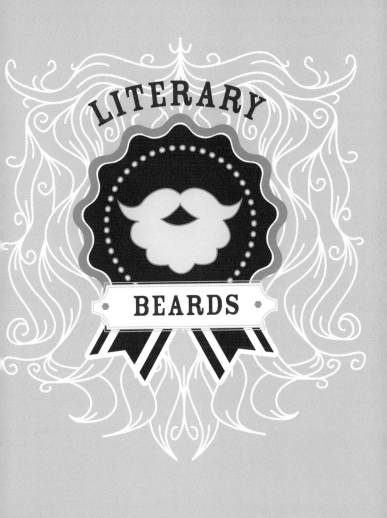

❧ JAMES JOYCE

Ah, James Joyce, author of *Ulysses*, the dirtiest book never to be banned in Ireland. When his father met James' future wife Nora Barnacle, all he could say was, 'At least she'll stick to you'. She no doubt said 'yes I will Yes' to the tache/goatee combo look he's sporting here.

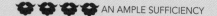 AN AMPLE SUFFICIENCY

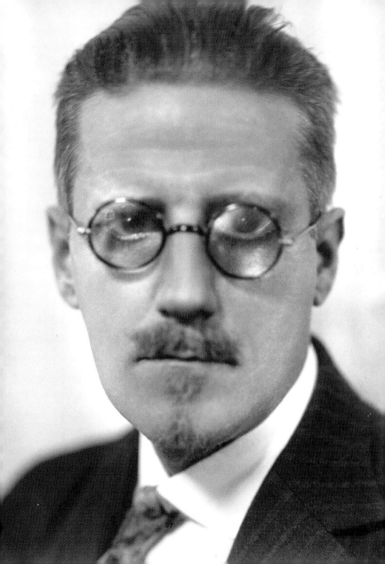

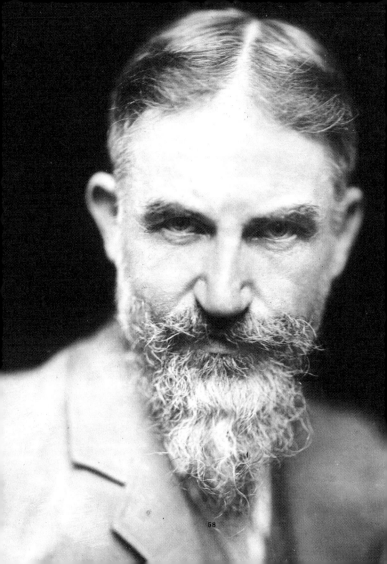

GEORGE BERNARD SHAW

Explaining why he had a beard, George Bernard Shaw told how, as a boy, he once asked his father why he shaved: 'He looked at me in silence, for a full minute, before throwing the razor out of the window, saying, "Why the hell do I?" He never did again.' And clearly, neither did GBS.

BEARD OF DISTINCTION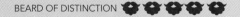

BRAM STOKER

Despite his incarnations on stage and screen, Clontarf native Bram Stoker's most famous character, Count Dracula is described in the book as, 'a tall old man, clean-shaven save for a long white moustache.' Perhaps Stoker had his own, luxuriant facial fuzz in mind when describing the world's most celebrated vampire.

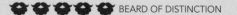 BEARD OF DISTINCTION

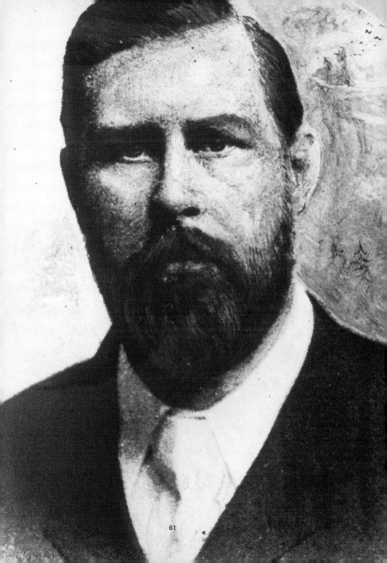

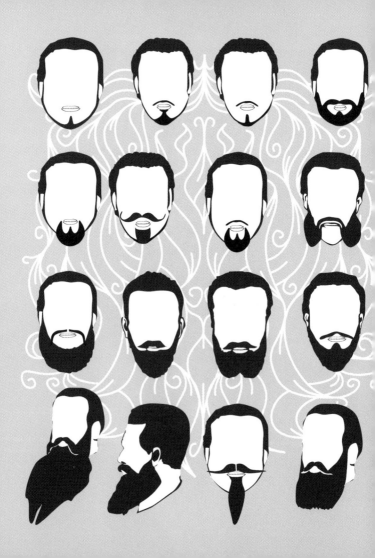

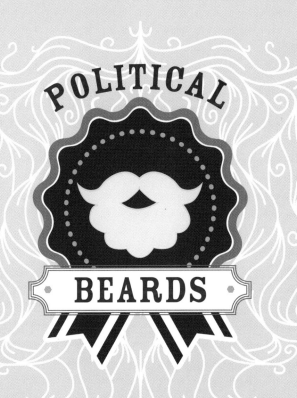

POLITICAL

BEARDS

☙ ROGER CASEMENT

This hero of the British Civil Service led a
chequered life and then lost his military honours
when he becamed involved in the fight for
Irish freedom. Still and all there's no denying he
was a snappy dresser, with the Victorian facial
accoutrements to match.

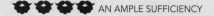 AN AMPLE SUFFICIENCY

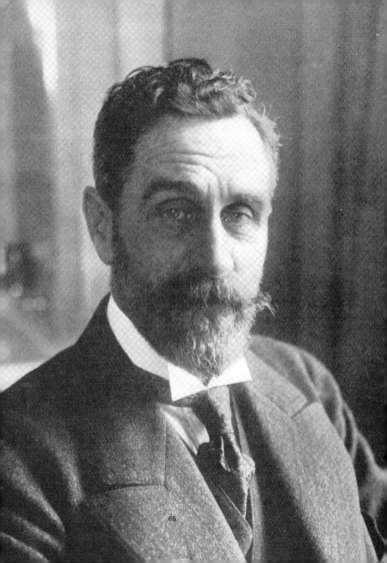

65

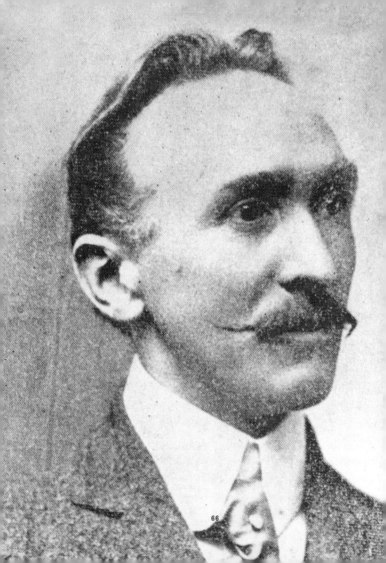

🐑 JOHN MacBRIDE

WB Yeats called this hero of the 1916 Rising 'A drunken, vainglorious lout'. Would a lout have the dedication to cultivate this fine specimen of nose-caterpillar? Never!

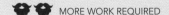 MORE WORK REQUIRED

WILLIE O'DEA

Was Willie O'Dea's most memorable moment when he posed with an automatic pistol aimed at a photographer? Or will he go down in the annals for featuring in the Rubberbandits' hit, 'Song for Willie O'Dea', with its immortal line, 'I swear by my tache 'tis daycent hash.'
Good man, Willie.

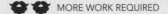 MORE WORK REQUIRED

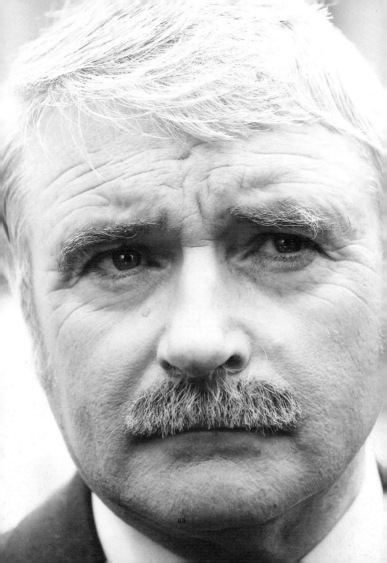

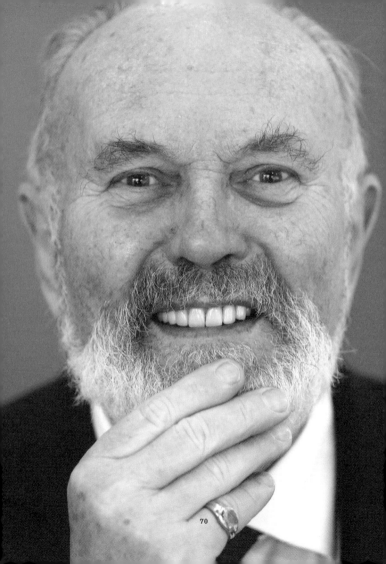

70

🐾 DAVID NORRIS

Scholar, senator and political activist, David
Norris is a founder of the Campaign for
Homosexual Law Reform. Did you know he is a
great practitioner of 'boxercise'? And as you can
see, the beard gets a workout too.

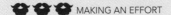 MAKING AN EFFORT

🐻 GERRY ADAMS

Between 1988 and 1994, the Sinn Fein leader's
voice was dubbed over in media broadcasts in
Britain and Ireland. At least we always got to see
his trademark glasses and beard. Indeed, rumour
has it Gerry was born with a beard; this rumour
has been neither confirmed or denied.

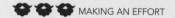 MAKING AN EFFORT

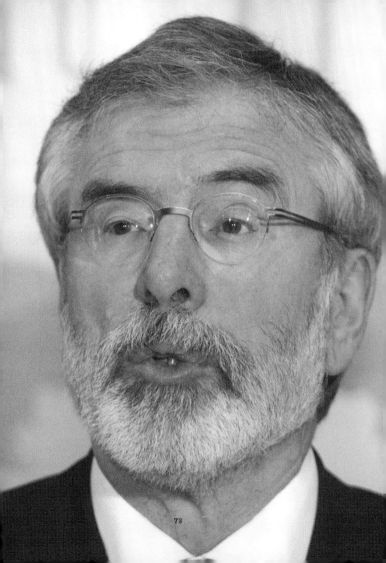

73

IMMORTALISE YOUR OWN BEARD HERE!

Beard of the Year Award goes to

● ●

For your services to facial hair we are truly
grateful. Go forth and grow!

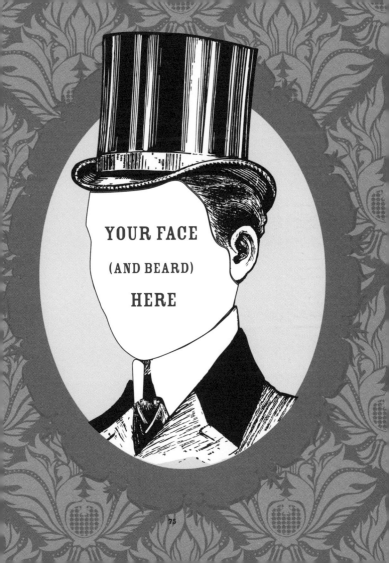

YOUR FACE

(AND BEARD)

HERE

BEARD ETIQUETTE

- If your chest hair meets your neck hair you are one lucky mofo – congrats on your magic carpet!
- When combing your beard, do so in a downward manner except on St Patrick's Day, when anything goes.
- A beard must be checked for food at least every fortnight, except in a leap year, when it should be checked weekly.
- If you find food in said beard, it is only ok to eat it if no one is looking.
- When two beards meet, the largest beard has right of way.
- When speaking about your beard, replace 'grey' with 'silver' and become instantly irresistible!
- So you're not the sharpest tool in the shed? Simply stroke your beard with one hand and nod sagely; you will immediately appear to be the silent, intelligent type.

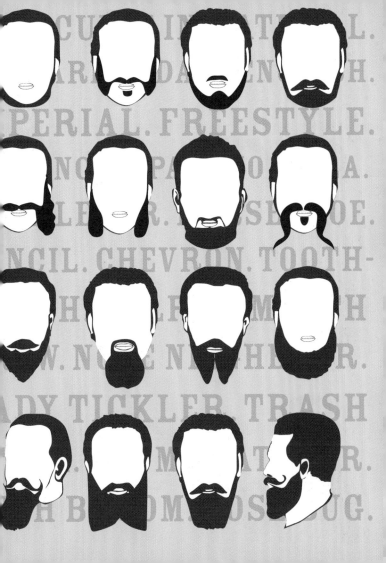

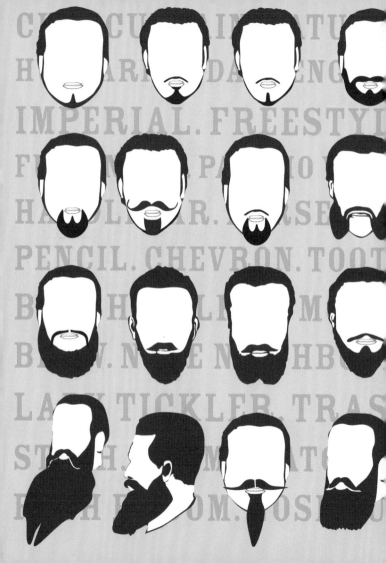